How I Lost 200 Pounds in One Day!

How I Lost 200 Pounds in One Day!

(And other fabulous things that happened when I became sick)

From the journals of

Sharon Henderson

To order additional copies of this book, contact:
Xlibris Corporation
1-888-795-4274
www.Xlibris.com
Orders@Xlibris.com
81560

Contents

*To Mom and Dad, who have always believed in me,
encouraged me to dream and loved me unconditionally.*

I love you both to the moon!

Foreword

IN THE WINTER of 2008, I was diagnosed with cancer and given only months to live. I then learned that instead, I had sarcoidosis, a rare and potentially fatal inflammatory disease that affects the organ systems of the body.

The initial cancer diagnosis came within days of when my youngest son, Chris, was involved in a near-fatal truck accident, the dissolution of my marriage and just two days before the birth of my youngest grandson, Landin.

Several months later, I began to keep a journal as a coping mechanism. I shared it with my mom, who forwarded it on to a few people. Over a few months' time, the e-mail list of those who received my journal entries grew and grew.

The journals helped me discover the blessings that came as a result of the illness and emotional upheaval of watching my son fight for his life.

This book is simply a compilation of some of the first two years' of journals. My hope is that the lessons and blessings I gathered along the way will somehow touch those who read it.

Chapter 1

On Love

I THINK IT was March 2008, but it might have been another month. Time around then blurred by, so I find I'm often short on details.

It was my first time sitting in the waiting room of this doctor – an oncologist, a cancer doctor. I wanted to discuss a biopsy, since I had been diagnosed with metastatic cancer. The doctors in Denver gave me a grim prognosis: Go ahead and go home, they said, there is nothing more we can do for you here.

They suggested that when I returned home to Gering, Nebraska, that I get in touch with oncology and schedule chemo and radiation, neither of which would cure me.

But for some reason, I decided I needed to know *exactly* what to call this cancer. The Denver doctor said the disease had spread everywhere. The doctors thought, perhaps, I had pancreatic cancer, since that's where they found the largest tumor. So there I sat . . . sitting, waiting, thinking.

The doctor finally walked in.

"So, why do you want a biopsy?" were the first words out of his mouth. "You already know you have cancer."

I replied, "Well, because I want to know which kind of cancer I have for sure. I want to know what to call it."

As we talked more, I told him that I wanted to treat the cancer naturally – the chemo and radiation scared me. I thought they might kill whatever good cells I had left. And besides, I explained, the naturopath whom I had talked to swore he could clean me up in 200 days.

The doctor looked me straight in the eye, put his hand on my shoulder and said, "Honey, you do not have 200 days."

That was then. This is now. We all know now that by some miracle, I don't have cancer. I have the inflammatory disease called sarcoidosis.

But for some unknown reason, God does not want me to forget the way this all started. He wants me to remember every detail: the diagnoses, the treatment options and talks, all of it. He wants me to never forget what it felt like thinking I had less than 200 days to live.

The feelings and emotions of this time still get to me. They still make me cry. I still feel raw and unprotected sometimes. Perhaps God wants me to feel everything so I can help someone else. Maybe He wants me to genuinely say, "I know just how you feel" when I try to comfort someone.

Or maybe He just wants me to appreciate what I have. But mostly, I think God wants me to understand that life is short.

He wants me to look at my parents and think, "They are not forever. Love them as such."

He wants me to look at my brother and sister and think, "They are not forever. Tell them how much you love them."

He wants me to look at my children and know that love is the best I have to offer them.

And He wants me to look at my friends and think the same.

And more than just *feeling* these emotions, He wants me to let them *know* what I am thinking.

So, I share my thoughts with my loved ones. I try to live my life as though I *really do* have less than 200 days. These good intentions are not as easy as you might think when it's hard crawling out of bed in the morning. But my goal is easier because I know I am doing everything to make love a priority in my life.

This goal has had its ups and downs. Mostly ups, but when you love someone who doesn't want to be loved, it's difficult. But I have learned something there, too.

I can still love those who don't want me to love them. I can love them on their terms and on my own terms, too.

There is someone in my life who refuses to let my love affect her. Oh, how it makes me so mad sometimes! But I know she wants to love. I know she wants to feel my love, too. I don't know why she can't. I hate that it makes me mad, but I am human.

So, I pray for her. I love her anyway. I get snarky with her sometimes, and it does me no good. So, I remember that life is too short to let someone's lack of ability to love affect my love for that person. And I go on.

My illness has been a driving force in my life – truly a turning point and a library of lessons that I'm learning as I go. The ability to share these lessons has healed me in many ways, and I thank each of you who reads this book for that.

The people I love and the way that I love them makes me the person I am. I am so blessed!

Chapter 2

A God Talk

KNOWING WHAT I know now, I probably have had the pain-in-the-rear disease of sarcoidosis since I was a young child. If learning about this disease followed the same stages as we grow in our lives, I would still be considered a newborn – maybe even an unborn!

This lack of understanding comes from the fact the sarcoidosis is mysterious and somewhat rare, having been discovered by the medical community only about 100 years ago. Plus, those of us who have this disease suffer from many and varying symptoms and side effects.

As I have written my journal, sarcoidosis has at least provided me with a topic! It's not the most pleasant subject, but my life is about nothing if not continually learning because of this disease. My friends and family have many questions about sarcoidosis that I haven't properly answered, and I hope this book will educate those I love while enhancing my own understanding.

In a recent discussion with fellow "sarc" sufferers, someone lamented that having sarcoidosis is like living with the flu every day for the rest of your life. That pretty much sums up my experience, as well.

Some days I feel sicker than others – *much* sicker. Some days I barely sense that anything is wrong. But yes, this feels like a perpetual case of the flu.

I sometimes wonder why God allows this type of crap to exist. I wondered so loudly, in fact, that God Himself apparently heard me, and we had a discussion that went something like this:

GOD: You are concerned about something? You can still bring it to me, you know!

ME: Oh, hi God. Yes, it has been a while. I haven't had a good heart-to-heart with you since when, last February or so? I'm still kind of ashamed about the bargaining thing I did.

GOD: Yes, that was the last time you came to me for help. I've been watching you though.

ME: I'm sorry, God. I'm so lost sometimes.

GOD: No, you're not lost. I've never let you out of my sight.

ME: Well, I *feel* lost sometimes.

GOD: I know, but if you remember that you don't have to do this alone, you wouldn't feel that way.

ME: I knew you were going to say that!

GOD *(chuckling)*: Yes, you did!

ME: I hate being sick. Why do you allow your children to go through shit like this? (Yes, I cussed to God. He didn't mind; He knows my heart.)

GOD *(laughing out loud this time)*: I sure have some forgetful children. Sharon, you know the answer to that question.

ME *(realizing immediately that I did know the answer)*: Oh yeah! It's the "path" thing, isn't it? *(I wanted to hit myself on the forehead V8 Juice-style just then.)*

GOD: You sometimes bury the knowledge that you have, child. Why?

ME: Because it's easier to blame you than me?

GOD: Gee, thanks! But yes, I know it's hard to look that deeply sometimes.

ME *(smiling)*: You know me well, Lord! So, it's about the lessons I'll learn, isn't it?

GOD: Not just *you*, but those you love and those who love you, too.

ME *(a little embarrassed)*: Ah, yes. I'm self-centered, aren't I?

GOD *(winking)*: Sometimes.

ME: Will I get to know the reasons in this lifetime?

GOD: Some of them, of course. But think of what you already know. Don't let yourself be blind to what you've already learned, child.

ME: I'm beginning to understand.

And so went our conversation about my inability to focus on the important parts and my need to forgive myself for my humanity. Suddenly, I knew that at least until God and I talk again, I would trudge along with little more knowledge and a lot more satisfaction in my soul.

I have learned one lesson for sure: My God has armed me with what I need to be strong and to allow myself to experience even the crappy parts of my life with some sense of knowing that it's not for nothing.

And that's how I handle life so far.

Chapter 3

Denial: It's Not Just a River

S INCE MY SARCOIDOSIS diagnosis in February 2008, I've become a relentless researcher of this disease. A self-proclaimed researcher, to be sure, but one nonetheless with Google as my new friend. When I learned I had the inflammatory disease, I spent countless hours learning more about it, trying to figure out just what the hell it is.

I learned a lot over the next eight months, but I am not sure if I've done a good job applying my knowledge. As I emerge from the denial about my disease, I am also learning to listen to my body.

I was terrified that I would let sarcoidosis, which is potentially fatal, claim me. Not claim my life, really, but my mind, will and ability to fight. I now find my illness much easier to accept and living with sarcoidosis comes more naturally. It's not like I have much of a choice!

My body now requires rest – *lots* of rest. My family understands this, but it's hard wrapping my mind around this some days. I tend to think I am letting my family down when I say, "I can't do this today," whether that means going to work, caring for my grandson, Noah, or even handling simple tasks.

I am so lucky I work for my family business. My family not only understands my need to rest, they encourage it. I feel shame in admitting this, but their understanding somehow makes me more determined to prove that I won't allow sarcoidosis to control my life – even if, in reality, it still does. Oh, how I *hate* that!

My powerlessness over my body frustrates me, and I don't want to allow myself to be sick. So, I deny it, but then I pay.

One day, God asked me about my denial. "How's that working out for you?" He asked.

And, damn it, I haven't answered Him yet. He pisses me off sometimes.

But God, you will be happy to know that I'm reflecting, and, I think, learning and growing. To answer your question, of course denial isn't working out for me well. I just want control over my body.

I stay grateful for each day, good and bad, even if I must answer to sarcoidosis before my life is over.

Chapter 4

Mad, Crazy Love

MY BOYS WERE 22 and 24 years when the house I had built was completed in October 2009. It happened at a time in all of our lives that allowed us to move in together. Coincidence? Hardly. I don't believe in coincidences anymore. I'm far more inclined to believe that God has a hand in every little event in my life.

When construction on our home started, I had talked to Aaron, my oldest, about moving in with my grandson, Noah. We decided to turn the basement into an apartment for them and that Aaron would rent it from me. It was a wonderful idea, and I'm so happy we did it.

Chris, my youngest, needed a place to live about the same time that the house was completed. I didn't have another apartment for rent, but I did have a large bedroom. So after a few negotiations, he was in, too.

It's uncommon for children their age to be willing to move home with Mom. But God has certainly blessed me with boys who love their momma. And I can't begin to thank Him enough for my relationship with them and for their willingness to be here with me when I need them so much.

The truth is, I didn't even realize how much I did needed Aaron and Chris – and it's not just for having men around for things I can't do.

Here's a story that shares the real reason I want them around so much.

One morning, I could hear Aaron and Chris downstairs puttering around as they prepared for work. This routine, in itself, always makes me smile. Even if I don't see them much during the day, just knowing they're around makes me so happy.

This particular morning, I heard Aaron say, "Hey, I love you, Brother."

The reply came a few seconds later: "I love you, too, Brother."

"Will you start my truck?" Aaron said.

"Yeah, I'll start it," Chris replied. "I'm on my way out now."

This is a small story, but it's nothing new because they have been close like this forever. This vignette also reminds me of another story.

When I still thought I had cancer that would kill me in less than 200 days, it crossed my mind that I would have nothing to leave my boys. I don't know why I worried about giving them a physical or monetary gift, but I thought about it for quite a while.

But the morning of Aaron and Chris's exchange, I realized something very important that makes me bawl my eyes out as I type this. I have already given those two boys everything they need for when I'm gone. They know the most important thing there is to know – how to love each other.

That's all they need, because their love for each other and for me is enough to build upon. This strong kind of love helps you love everything else that's important.

Aaron and Chris both have sons of their own now, and I know their love for their own children come from first loving each other. I certainly don't take full credit for their ability to love. My sons have had the best teachers in the world: their grandparents, aunts and uncles, extended family and their father. But I *will* take credit for a huge part of it. I'm selfish like that!

That day was important because I needed a reminder that Aaron and Chris don't wait for special occasions to say "I love you" and to help each other.

So no matter how badly I hurt, and no matter how stinkin' hard it is to walk down the stairs the first time each day, I will hardly even notice. God has reminded me of my own importance yet again. And if He's not careful, I'm going to get a big head! These things keep me going and make me strong.

I thank God for reminding me what I have to give and the blessings I've already received. I am, indeed, the luckiest person on the face of this earth.

Chapter 5

A Prayer Request

ONE DAY, A friend who also has sarcoidosis called. She asked how I was doing, touching base, etc. And, as she usually does, just before we exchanged good-byes she asked to please let her know how she could pray for me. I thought for a few seconds about what I needed and wanted most. Then it occurred to me: there are others who need prayer far more than I did. Let me tell you why.

Sarcoidosis has been around for a long time. Research reveals that this inflammatory disease is rather rare, but I don't believe it's rare at all. I think sarcoidosis is one of the world's most often misdiagnosed conditions.

For one thing, sarcoidosis mimics many other diseases, and that makes a proper diagnosis difficult. In my case, for instance, I was diagnosed with cancer – and not just treatable cancer, either. I was diagnosed with *terminal stage 4 cancer!*

Many of my "sarkie" friends have been diagnosed with cancer, too. Some were diagnosed with cancer first, then sarcoidosis later. Some were diagnosed with cancer in addition to sarcoidosis, which is something I worry about every day because it seems to happen quite often.

Others have been diagnosed with fibromyalgia, rheumatoid arthritis, chronic obstructive pulmonary disease (COPD) as well as various lung diseases, heart conditions and nerve disorders, just to name a few.

But, believe it or not, folks who have actually been diagnosed with *something* are the lucky ones. That's because there are hundreds of thousands of people out there (in my estimation) who can't even get a *wrong* diagnosis. They're told their ailments and miseries are in their heads. Why? First, *they don't look sick!* And second, their doctors can't pinpoint a diagnosis that makes sense and then won't revisit their findings.

Because I didn't have cancer, my sarcoidosis diagnosis thrilled my oncologist. I think, too, he wanted to work with a sarcoidosis patient. He asked if he could still be my doctor. He said he knew little about sarcoidosis, but that he was willing to learn.

At first, he seemed very happy that I took charge of my illness, researching it like crazy and learning right along with him. And then one day, I realized that I was learning more than he was. I was still learning, researching and gaining, and because he is an oncologist, I don't think he had any more time to invest in the learning process. He's an amazing doctor, but I think sarcoidosis was outside his expertise. He finally referred me to the doctors at National Jewish Hospital in Denver, for which I am very grateful.

Sarcoidosis is frustrating for those of us who have the disease, but I think it's also frustrating for doctors who don't understand it and can't confidently diagnose it. And maybe I give them too much credit. After hearing stories from *many* of my sarkie friends about poor treatment by doctors, I wonder if it's not just arrogance and a "could-give-a-crap" attitude that causes some to give up and leave us hanging.

So, instead of praying for my sarkie buddies and me, pray for our doctors. That's what I told my friend when she asked.

Pray for them to have patience with us while they sort out our many issues.

Pray for them to be gentle with us even in their frustrations, because they can't know the mental stress we face when they insinuate that our problems are in our heads.

Please pray for them to be lead to proper research so they can learn that sarcoidosis is not the disease described in outdated medical books: it strikes more than just 20- to 40-year-old African-American women; it's not just prevalent among people in the South; it's not just a lung disease. The research is out there.

There are sarcoidosis specialists now, and there are even huge hospitals that offer specialized sarcoidosis care. But sarcoidosis awareness obviously hasn't spread far enough.

So please join us in praying for these doctors so they can help us instead of making matters worse. And please pass this prayer request along to anyone who might help us pray and spread awareness. There are people dying worldwide because of doctors with no clue what sarcoidosis is.

Prayer is mighty, and I know all of you believe that. Thank you in advance for joining me and my friends – the brave, strong people committed to seeking answers and help and to getting our lives back!

Chapter 6

Superhero

AFTER I LEARNED I had sarcoidosis, I realized over time that my little symptoms were not so little anymore. That's when my skin began to hurt three or four times a week to the point it became painful to wear clothes.

I know that sounds nuts! Can you see the tabloid headlines now? "Woman crazed from disease becomes nudist against her family's wishes!" My skin burned and stung before, but never for very long – a few minutes to an hour or so at the max. But after a while, the skin pain was lengthy and horrid. The pain in my back worsened, too.

These ramblings make me feel pitiful! But they, in some way, stem from a "God talk" I had at that time. Let me share:

ME: God! I *hurt!*

GOD: I know you do. Why do you let things go for so long?

ME: What do you mean? I take my pain meds twice a day, right on schedule.

GOD: They haven't been helping for a few weeks now.

ME: They haven't? *(I can be pretty dense.)*

GOD *(laughing):* Well, have they? You take them every day. You rarely miss a dose. You still hurt. And you still cry.

ME: I think I'm just a wiener!

GOD: No, but you are awfully stubborn.

ME: True.

GOD: You think you deserve this. And you let things go.

ME: Not consciously, God.

GOD: True, but you do this. It bothers me. I've been waiting.

ME: I don't like my family to worry about me.

GOD: They do whether you say anything or not. In fact, they worry *more* when you don't say much.

ME: Huh?

GOD: They know you aren't in good health. They can see when you hurt. When you don't say anything, they worry.

ME: Oh, wow!

GOD: You have such great support around you. And did you know that some people's paths include dealing with you and your illness?

ME: *No!* Really?

GOD *(laughing):* Yes! It's not *all* about you! But you already knew that.

ME: I did. But I forget sometimes.

GOD: You are my human child. You are not perfect, and you are sometimes weak. It's OK to be weak. That's when you get the most help, and it's not always physical help, you know.

ME: God, you've given me much to think about, as usual. Thank you!

GOD: There are lessons to be learned in this, you know that. But you can be slowed by your own humanity. Just don't forget to let go sometimes.

ME: I won't, God. Thank you for loving me enough to be honest.

And on and on it went, until I fell asleep in the arms of my God as we talked into the night. Yes, God rocked me to sleep. It was wonderful!

I learned to be brave and ask for more from my doctor. Trying to be so strong makes me weaker in the long run. I'm starting to understand that old saying: "With God, all things are possible."

I'm a superhero – with sarcoidosis!

Chapter 7

Mom, This is for You

I COUNT MY blessings often. I may never write them all down, and I may not always voice a thank you. However, here's one story I gratefully share with everyone who will listen.

Mom, this is for you.

In my 45 years, no one has ever felt my pain like Mom. She has been there for me in so many ways, I'm not sure if I can write them all down.

My mom, Mary, and I shared a room at the St. Christopher House in Denver while my son, Chris, recovered in the hospital from an accident. That room was a sacred place for us. There was certainly nothing special about it physically, but if those four walls could talk, they would tell you that more tears were shed in that room in February 2008 than you could begin to imagine.

We cried for Chris. Sad tears followed by happy tears as he improved and recovered. And that's the room where we did *a lot* of crying for me.

I had been freshly diagnosed with cancer and given a pretty grim judgment. Mom was my pillar of strength during the day, every evening and many, many times in the middle of the night. We couldn't sleep very well in the room, so we talked. We cried a lot. We got pissed off, we got over it . . . and we laughed and laughed and cried some more.

That room in Denver is where my healing began, and it was Mom who led me to that spiritual place where God could begin my healing. I don't know if Mom realizes that, but I will never forget.

I lost track of the times I visited Denver hospitals for tests and appointments. Mom refused to ever let me go alone. She was by my side for every scary moment – for every required test, needle poke and painful grope that led to the horrid diagnosis of the dreaded "C" word.

And Mom was there when that diagnosis came. I thank God that Justin was there that day, too. I know that day was as hard or maybe even harder on Mom than me. But she refused to believe that I would die of cancer, and she stood strong in the face of some of the saddest news she had ever heard.

I know Mom didn't feel strong that day, but without her strength, I might have lain down and let a disease stake its claim on me without a fight.

There was ugly drama in my life that had nothing to do with cancer, sarcoidosis or Chris's accident. And because of Mom, I endured that as well.

My husband, Frank, was conspicuously missing during this time, sitting at home and refusing to see any seriousness in any situation. He missed me and felt sorry for himself. More about that later.

While we dealt with life without Frank, the reality of my marriage hit me like a ton of bricks as I lived in the little room at St. Christopher House. Mom's support gave me the strength to call my husband out and realize that he was holding me back. She supported me through my decision to end my marriage and to devote my energy toward my own healing rather than wasting it on a situation that would never change.

My entire family supported this decision, but Mom was there when I made it. She listened to me cry and wonder out loud if ending my marriage was the right course of action.

Thank you, Mom, for loving me the way you do. Thank you for trying so hard to understand this stupid disease and for your support as I sometimes struggle while learning more about what lies inside my body.

Thank you for your prayers and your belief in me, which helped me believe in myself. I could never repay you for the hours you have sat and waited, the time you have spent praying and hoping, the nights spent without sleep because of worry and fear. Please know that you helped me find the strength I needed to hang on.

If you're fortunate enough to have your mother here with you, hug her today. If you can't hug her, call her and tell her you love her. And if she is isn't with us anymore, share a "mom story" with someone you love!

Chapter 8

About the 'God Talks'

I ONCE HAD someone ask me if my conversations with God were real. I explained that yes, they are definitely real, and that I didn't feel special because God talks to me.

Some of you probably wonder about these "God talks" and how much of it I'm making up. Let me explain.

When my boys were very young and I was still married to their father, we became very involved in our Catholic church in Ogden, Utah. The priest for most of our years of attendance was Father William Flegge. Fr. Flegge was a wonderful teddy bear kind of man. Think Friar Tuck!

He's one of the wisest, most spiritual and wonderful people I have the pleasure of knowing. We shared many wonderful spiritual discussions and a soul-to-soul closeness that has played a huge role in forming who I am.

I believe that Fr. Flegge somehow knew my life's journey would require the knowledge he gave to me. And he shared his wisdom with a finesse that made every word stick in my memory. I seemed to file his words away so I could retrieve them at exactly the right time.

Fr. Flegge's relationship with God left me awestruck, and I told him so once. That's when he shared pieces of his life as we delved deeper into the subject of spirituality. He helped me realize I was responsible for hindering my relationship with God. It made sense when I understood my relationship with God should be easy, real, hopeful and close.

I also realized that my prayers don't need to be one-sided. That's when I started thinking about what would happen if I talked to God as if we were in the same room.

When I tried it, the most wonderful thing happened! God became present to me. My first conversation with God was definitely not one-sided, nor have any been one-sided since.

So, do I hear Him speak? I know that's your next question. The answer is yes, I hear Him!

As far as I know, nobody else hears Him when we talk, but I do – His words, His wisdom, His questions that I know are meant only for me. I see Him, too. I suppose it's in my mind's eye, but He's there. Even more than seeing Him, I feel His presence.

I should talk to God every day, but I don't. Only I limit our conversations. We talk whenever I initiate a conversation. And sometimes I wait too long to do so. But since I've been sick, we talk far more often. At first, I was ashamed at how far and few between our conversations were, but He knows my heart, and He knows what it took for me to return to Him.

Now those who know me understand that I am not a religious person at all. I don't attend church as often as I should, I don't talk about the Bible much and, as a rule, I don't "witness" to anyone.

But I have strong beliefs and convictions, and my relationship with God has made me aware of certain spiritual gifts I possess. I have learned that *anyone* can have conversations with God. *Anyone!* But He probably won't appear next to your bed one night and just start talking to you. You need to be ready for it, and you need to start the conversation with an open heart.

And then, you need to *listen!* I know that I'm not special – no more special than you. I also feel my type of God relationship isn't right for everyone else. And that's absolutely OK.

Because my conversations with God are ever present in my mind, my journals and this book have helped me put them on paper. So when I start to lose my mind, they will not be forgotten! I like to share the conversations once the lessons attached to them become clear.

This journey is a learning process. I am still unwrapping the gifts of my conversations with God, and the lessons He provides aren't always immediately clear. But I know they will be. He knows how I learn!

Chapter 9

My Noah

NEVER PRAY FOR patience! That's what Father Flegge used to say. When we pray for patience, we often don't realize the measure that God is willing to take to teach us to have it.

I prayed for patience once. Long before then, I was taught not to do so. God must have known how badly I needed to learn, because He's still sending me lessons that teach patience. One of those lessons is 5 years old, and his name is Noah!

Noah has taught me more than patience though, that's for sure. Because of my little Noah Sunshine, I have learned humbleness, persistence, the beauty of innocence and simplicity, true gratitude, hope and the need to fight with everything I have to overcome obstacles. But mostly, I have learned unconditional love. That's something I've always known, but to experience it together with your grandchild is right next to experiencing God.

Since I've been sick, I've spent a lot more time with my Noah. He doesn't really know that Grandma is sick, but he seems to understand that sometimes Grandma isn't quite right. He knows just when it's time to come and sit on Grandma's lap or crawl up in her bed and snuggle. And he doesn't ever get scared when Grandma sits and cries. That doesn't happen often, but Noah has seen this a few times.

He wipes my tears and says, "It's OK, Grandma." And he'll say, "Grandma, I have to tell you a question." This is always followed by, "You're my best friend I ever had in my world." Top *that!*

OK, he's not 100 percent angel. Darn close, but not quite. And some of those lessons he teaches me aren't just pure, sweet, easy-to-swallow lessons, either. For instance, have you ever tried to give medicine and eardrops to a 3-year-old convinced he didn't want them? I think everyone should try this at least once. The experience went something like this:

ME: Honey, we have to take medicine now. Grandma doesn't want you to hurt. Your medicine will help.

NOAH: No!

ME: C'mon, Noah, it will just take a few seconds. Let's hurry so we can watch that movie.

NOAH: I said *no*, Grandma!

ME *(a little perturbed now)*: Noah, you aren't the boss. Grandma is the boss.

NOAH: No, I'm the boss. *(You would think I would know this by now.)*

ME: Grandma has a surprise for you when you're done. *(Thinking quickly about what I have tucked away to give him.)*

NOAH: No, I don't want a prize.

ME: Noah, if you don't come and take your medicine like a big boy, I will have to force you to take it.

NOAH: *(silence)*

NOAH: *(I hear him running up the steps.)*

NOAH: *(I hear him running to his room.)*

ME: Dammit, Noah! I'm coming up there.

NOAH: *(silence)*

ME *(looking all over the place for Noah, finally hearing a tiny noise under my bed)*: Get out of there now, Noah! Come on!

NOAH: No!

ME: Fine! *(I put the red medicine on my desk and grabbed a little foot.)*

NOAH: No! No! No! *(Screaming now, crying, close to hysterics.)*

ME: *(I think I was actually growling like a pissed-off momma bear at this point.)*

That was the end of the dialogue. I picked him up, laid him on my bed right on top of a furry *white* blanket. I reached over and picked up the nice little cup of *red* medicine.

I'm thinking, how hard can this be? He's 3. I'm 43.

I held his arms together with one hand. (OK, who am I kidding? I had to practically lay on him to keep him still). I had one hand forcing his mouth open, the other ready to stick in the medicine. And would you believe that not one single drop of that *red* medicine went in his mouth. Every sticky, syrupy bit landed on that nice *white* blanket!

I cried. Not because of the mess, but from sheer frustration.

Noah stopped crying. Looking at me, he said, "Are you OK, Grandma?"

"I'm fine, Noah," I said. "I just don't want you to hurt. I'm going downstairs and getting more medicine. We have to try this again." Geez, I'm dumb.

So I got another cup of medicine.

Noah said, "I'm a big boy now, Grandma."

I'm thinking, "Great, he'll open his mouth for me," as I picked him up and prepared to lay him on the couch.

He started to throw a fit and said, "No, I'll take it myself."

So, I handed him the cup of red medicine against my better judgment. And he drank it down without another ounce of drama – or spilled red medicine.

Sigh.

Patience. Yep. I prayed for it.

I believe that God has sent me healing in the form of Noah. He has given me all the reason I need to never just lay down and let a silly disease control me. When Noah came to Earth, he brought with him magical, miraculous hope, healing and love to spread to every soul lucky enough to be part of his world.

I'm Grandma Sharon. I have hope, newfound patience . . . and sarcoidosis!

Chapter 10

Friendships

MY LIFE HAS been richly blessed with friends. I honestly can say a big bonus to moving frequently is the chance to make even more friends. I have been blessed with friends I carry with me in my heart, remaining close over the miles and years.

One friend in particular – a friend I thought I had lost track of – has been on my mind.

Jada lived across the street in Ogden when my sons were little. We met one day, instantly connected and began a wonderful friendship based upon genuine interest in each other and, eventually, genuine love. It's like we had known each other forever.

Jada helped me understand life from her unique and beautiful perspective and through her love of God. We talked about everything in the world, solved most of the world's problems and knew that life just didn't get much better. I missed her so much when we lost contact, like a part of me was truly empty without her. So it was no surprise that when we reconnected, we picked right up where we left off. Much had changed, but nothing had changed. We had the same friendship.

God puts people on our path knowing exactly how instrumental they will be in His design. Friends are gifts from God.

Let me tell you about my other best friends.

Carla

Carla is another beautiful sister I met living in Utah when the boys were little. One day, I called her, and she picked up the phone and said, "Hi, Sharon!" This was *long* before caller ID existed! Somehow she knew it was me – even though we hadn't talked like that before.

I loved Carla instantly. Our kids were friends; our husbands were friends; we bought a house in the cul-de-sac where they lived. We camped, ate, drank together, cried and prayed together so many times. Our friendship survived my divorce, my moving many times and hundreds of miles separating us.

To this day, Carla and I seem to have some psychic connection. I can sense when something is terribly wrong, and she seems to always call me when I need her most. Our lives have so many parallels that we almost expect it.

Mary

Mary and I are distant cousins whose friendship has trumped our "cousin-ship" many times over. We have had so many similar experiences that we understood each other from the word go.

Mary could relate to and understand my wilder side. She is the friend who makes me laugh until I hurt, who knows what I'm feeling when I lie and say I'm OK. She'll listen to some long, drawn-out explanation, look me in the eye and say, "OK, now the real story please." Yeah, that friend. I adore her!

Justin

Justin is just himself – a gift sent to me straight from the arms of Heaven when I was at my most vulnerable and didn't even know it. He stood by my side, held me, let me cry and led me through difficult times. He bargained with God for me.

He was there in the instant I heard some of the scariest news in my life and when I needed the strength to tell my husband not to be home when I arrived. He forced me to be honest with myself about my marriage. He was my live connection to someone in the other world I shamelessly miss every day.

Justin came into my life to save me from insanity. He told me that God wouldn't take me away from him so soon, so he knew that I would be OK. Besides my dad, Justin is the most selfless man I know. I can't imagine a world without him.

Susan

Susan and I have been friends since high school, sharing a bond that has kept our friendship special. We both were adopted as infants, have met our birth parents and understand each other from many different angles because of our similar lives.

We built our friendship on many memories and much laughter and still enjoy each other so much. I am grateful for Susan for so many reasons, and I hope she knows how special she is to me.

Kim

Kim and I have known each other since our boys were young. Our kids have been friends for as long, and we've shared many interesting and wonderful happenings. She makes me laugh, and we share similar hopes and dreams. She is the friend I dine with as often as possible, just to talk, laugh and share her company. I love Kim with all my heart!

Tricia

God put Tricia smack dab in my path to help me figure out parts of myself that I still didn't know even into my 40s. I relate to her beyond my heart – right into my soul. Tricia listens to every word, taking my every fear, hope and dream to heart and feels these emotions as I do. She helps me see myself so clearly, providing me encouragement and validation.

There are so many other friends not named here who have touched my life in wonderful ways. You know who you are, and I hope that I never leave any of you wondering how I feel. I love my friends, and I thank God for every one of you!

As I trudge along on my journey, I realized I have learned so much about myself and that each of my best friends helps define exactly who I am.

My strong hope is that your friends are those whom you can thank for helping you become who you are.

Chapter II

All the Stockings were Hung

IN PREPARING FOR Christmas in 2008, I got everything I needed done, despite my illness. Christmas tree? Check. Stockings? Check. Other home Christmas decorations? Check. Lights on tree? Check. Presents bought? At the last minute, check!

Everything was just right, but it was exhausting. I had to start then stop. I was just too tired to finish.

When I strung lighted garland up the staircase, it took a half-hour because I fought Benjamin (our adorable hell kitten) every step of the way. Winding garland shouldn't wipe out anyone, but I could have lain down and napped with no problem.

So, I decorated in streaks – working for a half-hour and resting for an hour. I call this "making concessions," and I decided to not be bummed about this. I'm thankful I was able to decorate for Christmas, regardless of how long it took.

About this time, I talked with the medical staff at National Jewish Hospital. The phone conversations were less than encouraging. The nurse told me it could take three months to be admitted.

But I had made up my mind: If it takes that long, then it's because there's a reason that I will deal with. I learned in 2008 that waiting isn't the worst thing to endure.

This experience, however, got me thinking . . .

Imagine standing on a street in a big city, waiting for someone to drop a few coins in your cup.

Imagine sitting in a nursing home, waiting for a family member, a friend – hell, just anyone – to come by and say hello.

Imagine waiting next to a loved one, knowing that he or she will cross over at any moment.

Imagine waiting for an organ transplant.

Waiting for a doctor's appointment is easy compared to any of these experiences. The realization hit me – I had nothing to complain about!

About this time of year more than 45 years ago, a woman waited.

Diane awaited the birth of her child.

The father of this baby had bailed. His family didn't know about the baby – and still doesn't know to this day.

There Diane sat, unwed and pregnant and facing an unacceptable station in life. Nothing was easy for her – neither her situation nor her decision to give her child a better chance. Quite honestly, I doubt much in Diane's life has been easy since. I don't presume to know her heart, but I've seen with my own eyes her life and the way her soul aches still.

After her child was born and given away for adoption, Diane began waiting again. This time, she waited for the day when her child would try to find her. After 34 years, that day finally came.

You see, Diane is my birth mother, and our meeting was the Christmas present my mom and dad gave me that year. They paid the adoption search fees so I could find my biological mother.

Mom and Dad did this, the most selfless gift I have ever known, for all three of their adopted children.

Meeting Diane was a healing gift to all of us: for me, my parents and for Diane. It was a happy time, but certainly not a "happily-ever-after" event. I lived with Diane for about four months so I could know her and learn more about myself, attempting to reconcile my past with my present and find peace. This experience was emotional and wonderful, horrid and eye opening. I walked away from this time with no regrets and grateful.

Grateful for Diane's 34 years of selflessness and for the life I was given with my adopted parents.

Grateful for the opportunity to get to know Diane.

Grateful that my life turned out the way it did.

I haven't talked to Diane in months. We don't keep in touch. I did call her to say that I had been diagnosed with cancer. She encouraged me, telling me that I was a goddess and reassuring me that I would be OK.

Then I called her two months later and told her that I didn't have cancer, but I had sarcoidosis instead. We talked for less than 10 minutes, and I haven't talked to her since.

I have reflected on why we didn't maintain a close and healthful relationship. I have reached an understanding, through the grace of God, which gives me peace about this.

I pray for Diane. I have hope for her. I want her to be happy and to experience joy every single day. That's because I know that Diane is still waiting.

I know that she loved me when I was born, and I know that she loves me still today, regardless of our inability to achieve a "happily ever after."

Chapter 12

Measuring

AS 2008 PASSED, I took stock of my blessings and the negative events of that eventful year. It's interesting to me that we humans put a timestamp on everything. God, of course, could care less about human time-markers. He simply gives us what we need when we need it, and life happens to us every moment. But we silly people need to measure time, our suffering, our grief – measure, measure, measure. This isn't always bad, but I've decided it's leaps and bounds better to measure positive events rather than the negative ones.

So when I look back on 2008, these are the blessings I measured.

In 2008, I was blessed . . . with learning in a few rather harsh ways that life is too short! It's too short to waste time on negative people. It's too short to worry about what others think. It's too short to spend precious moments trying to change people who never will. And it's too damn short to spend precious moments in the presence of anyone who can't see past the end of his or her own nose.

In 2008, I was blessed . . . with learning (again, rather harshly) that no matter how hard my life is at this moment, there is someone who has a much harder life; someone who has far more pain. There's always someone who has suffered loss and indescribable heartache that makes my own pale in comparison.

In 2008, I was blessed . . . to see first hand the strength of the human spirit in my family. I was blessed to experience the outpouring of love that comes with that kind of strength. Watching my family helpless, and frightened, waiting for answers, waiting for good news, waiting for miracles, I was blessed with hope, and my faith was renewed.

In 2008, I was blessed . . . with the gift of my son's near full recovery from a horrible truck accident. I was blessed throughout Chris's recovery with realizations about life, love, hope and faith. I was blessed by the outpouring of hope and prayers from friends and family. I was *so* blessed by the opportunity to be right there with Chris as he fought his way back to us – to hold him, touch him and love him through his own fears and frustrations.

In 2008, I was blessed . . . with a second baby grandson, little Landin Kooper Henderson. More light in my life, more love in my heart, and proof that just when you think you have felt the most love you can, you haven't.

In 2008, I was blessed . . . with many doctors who were caring, kind and willing to help me understand difficult procedures and diagnosis.

In 2008, I was blessed . . . with patience as I dealt with a diagnosis of a disease that nobody knows much about. But I was even more blessed by the friendships I made as I've researched sarcoidosis on my own, learning and growing in support with other people who have the same affliction.

In 2008, I was blessed . . . with a job that allowed me to be sick and away for so long during Chris's tragedy and my own illness while still paying and supporting me.

In 2008, I was blessed . . . that Mom had a sixth sense that told her I needed to get health insurance.

In 2008, I was blessed . . . with so many miracles I can't count them all. I am so grateful that I could experience them!

As each New Year dawns, some years will be harder than others, but *all* of them are a gift from God.

Chapter 13

Hope

MY LITTLE GRANDSON Landin's birth story is one you'd see on some reality TV program. To this day, it's hard to believe it's real. There's so much love and joy held in this story that I'm not sure if my words can do it justice.

Many of you know that when little Landin was born, his daddy was recovering in a Denver hospital from injuries received in a horrible truck accident. His mommy didn't know that we would be in Denver as long as we were with Chris and that her baby would be born in the middle of this chaos.

But that's exactly what happened. Little Landin was born in Denver on February 17, 2008, while Mommy and Daddy were parked side by side in identical hospital beds in a birthing room big enough to accommodate their unique situation. The staff set up a mirror so Chris could see Landin make his entrance, and he did his best to coach his wife from his bed.

A small group of us waited down the hall for a signal from someone that Landin was here. He gave that signal loud and clear all by himself when he screamed for the first time. I don't know how we avoided a flood of tears in that moment inside that little waiting room.

The previous few weeks had been such an emotional ride. So many scary, painful, horrific happenings, and here, in the middle of it all, a beautiful and wonderful event reminded us to hold on to hope. We still had so much to live for and work toward.

We took turns in the birthing room to see the beautiful boy. I don't know if I can accurately convey the emotions that commanded my mind and body as I held my new grandson for the first time. Given my illness, I wondered if I would be here to see him crawl, walk and talk. I prayed with every breath that I wouldn't get stuck being his guardian angel from Heaven.

Mind you, I have nothing against guardian angels – what an important and noble job that would be! But damn it, I wanted to chase his cute little butt around here on Earth and fulfill the job all Grandmas are supposed to do! I hated feeling sad when I should have felt nothing but pure joy.

Those moments helped me find my will to fight. I had so much to live for; I knew that I wasn't done yet. I knew that I would make count whatever days, months or years I had left. Even in the following months when I learned that I didn't have cancer and that my prognosis wasn't as grim as it once seemed, I knew I still had a mental and physical battle to fight.

I fight the battle to this day, but I am much stronger now. I am much more mentally able to keep my eye on what's important and what I have to live for. And I never forget how easily it all can be taken away.

Today, little Landin is a chubby-cheeked, blond-haired, blue-eyed firecracker who knows how much his "Mammaw" loves him. He is a constant reminder of how strong I need to be and how important it is to always keep hope in your heart.

Thank you, God, for the miracle of Landin!

Chapter 14

The Flight of My Soul

I DREAMED, ONCE again, that I could fly.

I'm never sad when I wake up from these dreams – it's more empowering than depressing. I think about these flying dreams for days afterwards.

When I dream, I easily thrust myself forward and upward, flying like Peter Pan or Tinker Bell or just some beautiful butterfly. In my dreams, I both see and feel myself fly.

The flying dreams seem to come when I'm feeling a little closed in, as if to remind myself that I am free – as unencumbered as I want to be. I think my dreams come from my soul.

I know my soul travels quite often as my body sleeps. It returns to me after spending time with those I love – both here and on the other side. When it comes back, I often feel renewed, comforted and made whole.

Sometimes, when I feel my body jolt in the night, it wakes me just enough to realize that my soul has returned to my body. The jolt makes me smile, because I know something beautiful just happened.

I then easily drift back to sleep knowing that nothing – not time, not distance, not even death – will ever separate me from the people I love.

Chapter 15

Thoughts on Love and the Lack Thereof

A S VALENTINE'S DAY in 2009 approached, I had more good health days than bad and more good days in a row than I had in months. I was almost afraid to say that fact out loud!

I had just a few issues with my heart rate – episodes of what I call "buzzy-ness." It's hard to explain, but I know this experience was related somehow to the sarcoidosis affecting my heart. I had random shooting pains that come with no warning, most often in my back and sometimes in my legs. They would hurt and then, thankfully, quickly dissipate. They came and went for a few hours at a time.

These pains are classic symptoms of sarcoidosis attacking my central nervous system. At this time, I was so looking forward to my visit to the National Jewish Hospital so the symptoms could be addressed more thoroughly.

During these weeks, I thought a lot about love. Maybe it was because Valentine's Day was just around the corner. You know . . . the "thanks-for-reminding-me-that-I'm-single" holiday.

I thought a lot during this time about the love that two people share. The kind of love Mom and Dad (my heroes!) have shared for 50 years. The love that was absent in my relationship with Frank, even after nine years together. And thinking about that relationship made me think about how we settle for less, just to have something.

Not everyone does this, of course, but I do know plenty of people who have and still do.

And then there's me. I obviously did it. I've talked to God about this many times. And I'm finally satisfied with the answer that I knew I would receive from Him.

The answer, of course, is that we all learn during our life's travels. And, of course, my nine-year journey with a lame-ass dud by my side taught me many wonderful lessons – some I haven't fully realized yet, without a doubt.

It's tempting to consider all of that time a waste, but I know better. And I knew I needed to talk it over with God to sort through everything properly.

In hindsight, my reasoning was simple. I wanted what every woman I know wants: to be loved and accepted for the person that I am. And let me tell you, some people are really good at convincing you that this is what's happening when it's not.

But the truth lies somewhere in the chaos your life becomes when the relationship ends. The truth in my case lay so distant from what I had hoped that it's almost embarrassing to think I fell for it.

Believe it or not, I still haven't given up on the idea that there's someone for me. I still believe in miracles, and I completely and unequivocally believe in love. Am I crazy? Probably. But I can't help myself. Sometimes, hope and faith is all we have. I can't imagine not having either one of them.

Chapter 16

How I Lost 200 Pounds in One Day!

TRUTH IS STRANGER than fiction, they say. That's what I tell myself when I think about the end of my marriage to my second husband.

In November 2008, Frank, my boyfriend of nine years, and I tied the knot. My family wasn't crazy about the idea – because they weren't blind like I apparently was! But they supported me anyway, giving me yet another reason to adore them all.

My wedding (affectionately labeled "My Big Fake Wedding" by my dear friend, Mary) took place in Colorado just three months before Chris's accident and my health diagnosis.

The day after Christopher's truck accident, we learned he would be transported to Denver because they just couldn't fix him at the hospital in Scottsbluff. I knew immediately that I would go to Denver to be with Chris, and I assumed that my husband would either come along or follow shortly. Turns out, I couldn't have been more wrong.

Frank told me he didn't think he could stand to see Chris "that way" and said he would be more useful at home. I kind of understood where he was coming from, but not knowing the full extent of Chris's injuries, I wasn't sure how long I would be gone. Plus, there really wasn't anything at home more important than supporting my son.

I was too stressed to argue the matter, and I didn't need to be at odds with my husband with everything else going on. So I packed my bags and left for Denver with my mom.

Chris didn't do well on the ride to Denver. His broken femur triggered a fat embolism, which caused respiratory failure twice before he arrived in Denver and once more immediately after the arrived at the hospital. Because Chris was in traction, his doctors thought it would be too difficult to load and unload him the extra times that would be involved had he been flown.

Within two hours after we arrived in Denver, doctors told us Chris might not make it. As a last-ditch effort, the doctors laid him prone to force his lungs to fill with oxygen. They told us that if this strategy worked, it would work immediately. But if it didn't, there wasn't anything else they could do.

We went to the trauma unit to see Chris, not knowing if this would be the last time I would see him alive.

That's when I bargained with God. I told Him, "Let Chris live, and I will take anything You have to give me!"

I already knew I probably had cancer. Just two days earlier, my CT scan showed nodes that were likely cancerous, but I couldn't even worry about that. I just wanted Chris to live.

I bargained with God for what seemed like hours, even though I knew better – and even though I understood in my heart that's not how life works. Just 20 minutes later, one of Chris's doctors came out to tell us that the procedure had worked. His lungs had immediately filled. He was alive!

He would need to stay prone for 24 hours, and they told us that we probably wouldn't recognize him when they turned him over. But I didn't care. I knew that no matter what else happened, my son was going to live.

We stayed in Denver for nearly a month. During that time, I decided on further testing to see exactly what was wrong with me. After several tests, I received the diagnosis: stage IV metastatic cancer.

After every test, I called Frank with the latest updates. He never really seemed to accept that my medical condition was very bad. He would say make comments like, "Well, that's not so bad. People live through these things all the time."

He didn't seem to process anything I said. He would call me and refuse to talk about my situation. I would beg him to come to Denver for my next tests, and he had every excuse in the book. He seemed to be pulling further and further away from me when I needed him the most.

At first, I made excuses for Frank. It must be difficult for him, I told myself. I told everyone who asked that he was "holding down the fort," even though I felt like an idiot knowing that the people who loved me saw through the excuses I made for him.

After begging Frank to come from Gering to Denver for the weekend (it's a three-hour drive) for the third time, I just couldn't deal with his excuses anymore.

I called him later that night and told him I needed to talk. He said I sounded angry and wanted to know why.

"I am sick of your excuses," I told him. "I don't understand why you won't or can't be here for me."

And this man – the man I had married, the man I had known for more than nine years – replied, "Well, what about me? You know how I hate to be alone, and you have left me here all alone. How do you think I feel? How could you do that to me?"

Yep, he said that. Exactly like that. And the only words that would come out of my mouth were, "Please, don't be there when I get home."

Of course, Frank was appalled, inconsolable and kept saying, "What? I don't understand what I did. What?" But he had said all he needed to say. I was done.

No one in my family was surprised. Go figure! Finally, my blinders had come off. I ignored so many things over the years because I loved him, but this was truly the straw that broke the camel's back.

This story also has an interesting postscript: It turned out that my marriage wasn't exactly what I thought. Our marriage was never recorded by the State of Colorado, making it nonexistent.

So, we didn't even go through a divorce, which I guess was lucky for Frank. He had left for another state with his new girlfriend shortly after I returned from Denver. I understand they were married not long after that. You do the math . . . it hurts my head!

And that, my friends, is what I mean when I say I lost 200 pounds in one day!

Chapter 17

Random Me

I'M A PHOTOGRAPHER, graphic designer, writer, reader, grandma, momma and friend. I am many things; I am me.

I believe in God. I talk to Him. He answers me. I don't care if you think I'm crazy. I'm a little insecure. I'm OK with that. I'm strong. I'm weak. I'm real. I love life as a grandma, just like I love life as a mom. I want bunches of grandkids. Bunches! I feel younger than I am. I love to laugh. I need to laugh. I'm genuine. I'm bitchy. I'm happy. I love my life. A lot!

I'm purple, and I'm green. I love potatoes. I don't require a lot of sleep. I love to write. I love to talk. I enjoy conversations with substance.

I spend too much time on the computer. I daydream. I work. I get up early. I go to bed late. I don't watch the boob tube much. I read a lot.

I love to hear my grandkids say, "Mammaw?" I love to see them communicate in their own way.

I have sarcoidosis. I have hope. Lots of it.

I am peanut butter and macaroni and cheese, but not together.

I dislike shopping most of the time. I think pizza is OK, but I'm not crazy about it.

I love to learn. I think I could be a professional student.
I play the piano. I sing. Not very well mind you.
My eyes are greenish. My hair is curly.
I love weird words. I love purses. I love sweatshirts with hoods.
I love blue jeans and flip-flops.

I love quirky people and people who have something to say – and not just with
their words. I love to listen.

I'm a people watcher.
I love animals. New socks are fabulous.
I turn the music up in my truck and sing like nobody can hear me.
I need the mountains. I don't drink milk.

If you can make me laugh, you can own my heart!

Chapter 18

Tools

GETTING "UP CLOSE and personal" with myself has been a big challenge, and possibly my biggest accomplishment, since I've been sick. There's nothing quite like having your body, soul and spirit immersed in a disease to make you look long and hard at who you really are.

I think the process involves self-preservation. We attempt to figure out who we are so we can persevere; so we can stay one step ahead of difficulty; so we can be at peace; so we can simply be.

Before I became sick, I ignored who I was. Not on purpose, of course; it's just how I lived my life. I thought I knew what was expected of me as a wife, mother, daughter, sibling and friend. I lived my life for everyone but myself.

I was happy to do that, because it had never occurred to me that life could, or should, be any different. I convinced myself that I was happy. I tolerated crappy behavior from people who, had they loved me, would never have treated me that way. I excused their behavior to myself and to others.

Looking back on that time in my life, I can see pretty clearly that, somewhere in my soul, I knew I was wrong. Somewhere sleeping deeply inside of me was a love for myself that today would *never* allow me to happily accept such things. I grew into a different person because I was forced to examine who I was.

Unhealthy relationships with men – none of which included the familial relationships with my dad, brother and sons – taught me some of life's biggest lessons.

I married one of these men. I "married" another ("my big fake wedding") and lived with a third. The sum total of these three men in years comes to 24 or so. The temptation is to look at these years as a waste of time, energy and mental health.

But I know differently now. It turns out they were *all tools!* (Oh, I crack myself up!) OK, so they are tools, but they are tools of God! And it turns out I'm not such an easy child to teach, so He allowed me to keep changing tools to help me get it right.

The lesson to be learned is that God uses the people He puts in our life to help us to become the child He had in mind when He created us. The seemingly unfortunate events we live through with some of the worst people we know make us stronger – and ultimately happier – people.

We all need tools to fix things and create things. God uses tools, too, and we don't get to doubt His reasons. If we learn from the mistakes we make, if we become better, stronger people, then in the end, there are no mistakes.

Chapter 19

The New 'Normal'

AS SPRING 2009 approached, I had been treated to sunshine, warm days and feeling good health-wise. For the first time in a long time, I had felt (gulp!) like my old self. It had been so long that I often wondered if I would know what feeling good was like. It turns out that I did know, but it's not quite the same as before my illness.

For far too many years, I took feeling normal for granted. I never gave a second thought to how it might feel to be unhealthy. Hell, I never gave it a *first* thought!

I think humans naturally take a lot for granted, living our ordinary existences. We fall into comfortable routines and then life suddenly changes and *nothing* feels normal, at least for a while.

And if we're really lucky, nothing's normal again. Lucky, you ask? Yes! I've learned that if I had always been "normal" and had never gotten sick and had never had new experiences because of my illness, there are many lessons I would have never known.

I wouldn't have known the feeling of telling my sons that my most recent tests were back and that the results weren't so good. Not a peachy day for sure, but I wouldn't have experienced their reaction otherwise – a memory I still have today.

The day you realize you may not have much time with the people you love is the day that changes everything. *Everything!* If you thought you had the strongest love on Earth for your children, and that you couldn't possibly feel a greater love any more fully, you'll learn that you were wrong.

You'll never hear certain words in the same way, such as "my mom/dad/ brother/sister/aunt/cousin has cancer."

Your gut ties up in knots for them. When you've been in that scary and unpredictable spot, you don't just hear the words, you feel that pain, that terror. And when you tell them you're sorry, they *know* you understand. That understanding becomes a gift.

You will never see certain things in the same way, either. In the midst of the chaos, I held my second grandson, Landin, in the days after he was born, not knowing if I'd see his first steps and get to know him and watch him grow. Those thoughts made me very sad, but I started looking at him differently, too. I appreciated every moment spent with him in my arms, every breath he took, every baby noise made by his tiny body. I saw more than a child; I saw an absolute miracle.

When my oldest grandson, Noah, came to see his new little cousin, it was the first time in a few weeks I had seen him. My heart broke into a million pieces as I hoped with everything in me that I had somehow been able to make enough of an impression on his little life so he would always remember me.

That's when it suddenly became a driving force to make a difference in the lives of my loved ones. Other than with my grandsons, who were so young, I wasn't afraid of being forgotten. But I quickly realized my family members needed to know how much I loved them. These were thoughts I couldn't just *tell* them. I had to *show* them.

About that time, I lost my tolerance for people, especially those connected to my family, who want to play games and create ridiculous, unnecessary drama. It's that whole "life is too short" attitude. When faced with the possibility that your life might be cut short, you gain insight into the lives of the people you love. It becomes difficult to watch them waste their time with situations that clearly won't change.

I wanted, I think, to make sure they weren't stuck in unhappiness when I couldn't help them through it. Yes, I know it's ridiculous to think you can protect those you love from life's circumstances, but it doesn't stop you from wanting to get *your* life in order as well as theirs.

Life becomes funnier, and you become more willing to look ridiculous while laughing at them until you cry or hurt. Time becomes more precious, and you become less willing to allow the tasks of day-to-day life to interfere with worthwhile things. And "worthwhile things" suddenly have less to do with financial or material gains and far more with filling your spiritual bucket.

You learn that relying on God makes you strong, not weak. You become more willing to listen more intently to His voice and more willing to remain still to feel His touch.

And, somehow, your life becomes not your own. You begin to see the value in sharing your life completely, spreading your gifts as far as you can among the people you love and gathering along the way important gifts to take with you.

You do this not because you're concerned that your life isn't worth remembering, but because you want the people you love to experience the life made possible only when "normal" is just a word in the dictionary.

Be certain that whatever must happen in your life to kick-start your journey is absolutely worth the pain.

Chapter 20

Humility

THE PRAYERS AND healing vibes from everyone have been a true blessing as I have dealt with my sarcoidosis. These prayers help every time I deal with the not-so-pleasant aspects of dealing with sarcoidosis, of which there are many. But once again, this disease has brought about many blessings and opportunities that I otherwise would never have known.

At one point during my treatment in Denver, I returned for more testing, which included two MRIs, an EMG test (an electrical study of my heart, basically) and a visit with my new heart doctor. This one day of testing was worse than the three days' worth I had three weeks earlier. But I survived and am probably now stronger because of it. With all of the holes they poked in me, I probably was leaking something and didn't even know it!

Here is the account of my treatment that I wrote at the time:

I returned to the National Jewish Hospital in Denver on June 26 for an electromyogram (EMG), an electrical study of my heart. If they find any scarring whatsoever during this heart catheterization, they will implant a defibrillator. But the doctor seemed fairly optimistic that this wasn't necessary, based upon the heart MRI and PET scan I had a few weeks prior. This is *great* news!

The studies show that sarcoidosis has inflamed my heart, and inflammation comes before the more-damaging scarring stage. We want to avoid this, obviously, so barring any unforeseen discoveries in the electrical study, I will begin a stronger medicinal attack on the sarcoid. The PET scan also showed other areas of sarcoid that I hoped wouldn't be there. But in reality, I'm wasn't that surprised.

I came home this time with much more information. And after speaking with the doctors, I know at least that there's a plan in the works.

My experience as a "lab rat" taught me a bit about humility, a quality that's important to learn during our time on this planet. Trust me when I say that humility lessons are not glamorous.

I've spent more hours than I care to count wearing fabulous hospital gowns parading in front of strangers as I try to look adorable. (Just kidding about the adorable part. After a while, you just don't give a crap about how you look; you just want the tests to be *over!*)

I especially love the way the technicians size you up, trying to decide if you need a normal-sized gown or the specialty elephant size that they sometimes toss your way. Thankfully, I could wear normal-sized gowns. But apparently some of the techs weren't too sure, and a few times I walked down the "lab rat runway" wearing a tent. Fabulous, I tell you!

The medical world has some new fashions, and last week, I modeled one – a pair of lovely blue *paper* shorts. Mom wanted to photograph my "absolutely stunning" medical wear, but I didn't want to make you all jealous. The generous doctor told me I could take them home, but I would struggle to find a top to match such lovely things, so I left them behind. My pride knows no bounds.

Early in life, I discovered that I'm not blessed with cooperative veins. When I visit the lab, it's never quick and painless. My veins are tiny, and they roll, blow or just plain disappear almost every time I have blood drawn or an IV started.

When I had four MRIs recently, the pain was especially horrible. After being poked four times without any luck, "Nurse Ratched" came in to save the day. She finally decided to stick me on the underside of my wrist – somewhere I had never been poked because *most* people don't want to put you through that kind of pain. I screamed some choice words – very loudly!

Mom sat in the waiting area the whole time and, thank goodness, didn't hear me. She would have freaked out. Still, I came out crying – that's how badly it hurt. And, keep in mind, that I'm a tough cookie.

I've been poked, prodded and hurt many times and have never shed a tear, but this session truly hurt like hell! In Nurse Ratched's defense, she kept saying, "I'm so sorry, I'm really sorry" the whole time she jabbed me, but I was still mad at her a week later. At any rate, the lesson learned here is all about humility and trust.

Reading the National Jewish Hospital doctors' dictation notes can be humbling, too. Not only do they write about your illness, they write about what they think of you. Fortunately, no one thinks I'm a hypochondriac, which is how I felt before I went there even though all of my tests showed horrible things.

Especially interesting were the eye-opening comments about how I "appear" or "seem." Apparently, I still have a "moon face" from the drug Prednisone, which was far worse three months earlier. The side effects of Prednisone suck; I hate them.

Reading how extensive my disease appears to the specialists is also unnerving. But reading the notes let me know that we're headed toward new treatment frontiers. The doctor thankfully listened when I told her that I don't tolerate steroids well. So it's looking like chemotherapy drugs for me, which I know have side effects – and not very pretty ones – all of their own. But if the side effects don't make me want to crawl out of my skin, that will be a bonus.

I've made my peace with the possibility of losing my hair. Hopefully, the doses won't be strong enough to cause that, but it could happen. I love my hair, but I'd love to feel normal again far more than that.

It sucks that I must make that choice. But you know, I'm pretty damn grateful that I *have* choices.

Chapter 21

Out with the Old

THE LAST NIGHT of 2009 went out with a bang – not an exclamation point to punctuate the year, but more like a thundering voice from above pronouncing, *"Hold up, Kiddo. You still have something to learn!"*

That's because I received a long-awaited phone call the evening before bearing a message I could have waited much longer to hear. My cardiologist had called me personally, which made the hair on the back of my neck stand straight up and fast.

He told me that the Holter monitor he had me wear for 24 hours two weeks earlier showed that my heart had demonstrated episodes of ventricular tachycardia (V-tach). It was time, he said, to get a defibrillator (called an AICD) as soon as possible.

After spending all afternoon on the phone with both National Jewish Hospital and University Hospital in Denver, my AICD implantation surgery was scheduled for January 4. All things considered, this was a good way to start the New Year – with peace of mind. There's no price you can put on that, is there? A defibrillator can save my life, and that's how I chose to look at it. But to say I wasn't scared would be a big, fat lie.

Here is what I wrote after I learned I needed the defibrillator:

I'm not sure what lesson I have to learn from this yet, but I do know there will be one. There always is. I also received a phone call today from Dr. Gottschall, my chief sarcoidosis doctor. She told me the tests I had two weeks ago show no improvement in the sarcoid compared to six months ago.

She started to tell me to up my methotrexate (an autoimmune drug) now, but she hadn't heard the "big bang" news yet, so she told me to "scratch that" and that she would get back to me next week after the defibrillator is implanted.

So, that's the report I waited so long to hear. (Two weeks is *long* when you're me!) I honestly thought that because the results took so long, that "no news is good news," but that is not always the case. Don't believe it when someone tries to tell you that!

But there's still hope. Lots of it. The sarcoid isn't getting worse, but it's not responding well to the current treatment. If the sarcoidosis wasn't wreaking havoc on my heart, it would be tempting to just live with it. But that's not smart either, considering that the longer the inflammation is present, the more it will damage the organs that host the disease.

I promised my cardiologist that I would take it easy and stay low key until Tuesday. My children have confined me to the loft! The upside is they have to wait on me hand and foot – even if I'm a fairly low maintenance prisoner. The downside is that there will be no big New Year's Eve party here tonight as we had originally planned. That's OK with me though; I'm scared enough to do pretty much nothing right now.

I promised Dr. Buckner, my cardiac sarcoidosis specialist, that I would not drive alone and that someone would stay with me until I get there. So, New Year's Eve at my house will be spent up here in the loft.

I'm pretty sure we have some champagne and a few board games to ring in 2010. Maybe even a few episodes of "The Big Bang Theory, Season 2." Seems appropriate doesn't it?

Chapter 22

Heart for My Heart

I'VE NEVER THOUGHT about my heart in the same way since January 4, 2010.

That's when I became the proud, happy owner of a defibrillator, a mechanical device (that I've named Thumper) designed to stand guard over my heart and its quirky, speeding ventricular tachycardia. Thumper is a pocket watch-sized computerized peace of mind packed with a bit of goodness. Once again, I'm blessed beyond measure.

The implantation of Thumper went exactly as expected. There were no surprises or abnormalities, and I stayed in the hospital exactly as long as they said I would. I have a scar on my chest that's about 2½-3 inches long. Seeing that scar, and knowing what lies just beneath, gives me comfort that I can't explain.

When I left the hospital the next afternoon, I sat on a couch in the lobby while Dad retrieved the car from the valet and Mom filled my prescriptions at the hospital pharmacy. A lady came around with a coffee cart, offering hot coffee to those waiting for family members and people wandering around watching it snow outside.

As she walked closer to me, I noticed a young man approaching her to get a cup of java, pulling around an IV pole with five or six bags full of fluids pumping into his body. He was so glad to get that coffee that I jokingly said, "Hey, you should see if she can just pour coffee in one of those bags!" The young man laughed, and we struck up a conversation.

I never did learn his name, nor he mine, but our conversation was like we had been friends our entire lives. He told me he was on a waiting list to be placed on a waiting list for a lung transplant. Can you imagine . . . a list to get on a list?

I told him, "Dude, that sucks. I'm so sorry."

"Oh, don't be," he replied. "I'm at peace with whatever happens."

Looking at him, I knew his matter-of-fact statement was true. He talked about the blessing of his family's support, something I could relate to without question. We discussed sarcoidosis a bit, and we also learned that we were both at University Hospital in Denver for procedures, but that our main hospital was Denver's National Jewish.

"Hey! We have something else in common," he said. "Our disease names rhyme!"

We laughed so hard about that – he has cystic fibrosis; I have sarcoidosis.

I doubt you laughed at that little joke just now. But to us, that comment was so goofy and funny. When Dad returned with the car at the same time Mom showed up with the prescriptions, I felt I had been given 20 minutes with an angel from Heaven.

God did that. He gave me Thumper, to take care of my heart physically, and He gave me time with that angel, to take care of my heart spiritually. He gave me heart for my heart – just when He knew I needed it.

I will never forget that angel and that conversation. I doubt I'll see this young man again, but he was a gift that I gratefully unwrapped.

Are you sick and tired yet of reading about how blessed I am? I never grow weary of telling you all. I am *blessed* so immensely that there aren't enough words in all of the thesauruses and dictionaries to make sense of it.

I am one loved girl!

Chapter 23

And Along Comes Princess Pink

MY FAMILY IS pretty good at producing little boys: I have two sons; my sister has two; and my brother has three. That means my parents have seven grandsons!

And then when my boys started having babies, they were boys, too. Somewhere along the line, we stopped dreaming about cute little frilly pink things, and thanked our lucky stars that we didn't have little girl drama to deal with. (That was sour grapes, you know!)

So imagine our surprise when Nichole, my daughter-in-law, has her first ultrasound with her and Christopher's second baby and the doctor tried to tell us it was a girl.

Riiight! We don't have girls in our family anymore. Wait, what? Are you serious? I think they had to reassure Nikki on three different ultrasound occasions that the baby indeed lacked little boy parts. Personally, I only needed to hear that once before I bought my first little pink pair of socks. After the second ultrasound, I'm not sure what came over me. I had pink fever!

So just about 3½ weeks before her actual due date, our tiny and beautiful Addlee Laine Henderson made her debut into our family on April 9, 2010. She was so much smaller than the boys were, partly because she was a little early. And, I think, partly because she's just a petite little princess!

I admit to, at first, freaking out a teensy bit. You wouldn't think there's a lot of difference between her 5 pounds 2 ounces and her brother's 6 pounds and change or her cousin Noah's 7 pounds and a few ounces.

But there was. She looked smaller; she felt smaller. And I wasn't at all sure how adeptly I could hold her. But that feeling melted away the second her mommy put her in my arms.

I'd done all of this before, but I've learned that each new grandbaby is like getting a brand new gift from God. All visions of pink and frilly things aside, I fell in love all over again. Memories of me with my grandma came flooding in, and I knew that little "Princess Pink" and her "Mammaw" would have a very special relationship, too.

And again, I am so incredibly blessed!

Chapter 24

The Rules

THESE ARE MY rules – lessons learned that I hope to live by.

1.   **Family is not where bridges should be burned.** Regardless of how angry you are, and how right you think you are, it just doesn't matter if there is family love at stake. *Always* reconsider when you're tempted to write off a family member.
2.   **A genuine relationship with God is more important than following the rules of a religion.** Talk to God as if He were sitting right next to you. No, this doesn't make you a candidate for the psych ward.
3.   **People change.** Sometimes they change for the better; sometimes, not so much.
4.   **Children can teach you.** This happens once you forget that you aren't always right just because you're an adult.
5.   **You don't get to choose the way that people love you.** You don't control much of anything. Sometimes love is a choice that you have to make every morning when you wake up.
6.   **Life often is easier than we think.** When life starts to seem hard, it may be time to re-evaluate it.
7.   **The most important gift you give your children is your time.**

8. **You can never take back words you say.** Once they are said, the damage is done. Think twice before you speak those words if they aren't words of love.

9. **It is an absolute *must* to find humor in your life every day.** Life is too short to live otherwise.

10. **Love is the most important thing.** *Always!*